Smell No More

A Do It Yourself Guide On

How To Stop Smelly Feet.

Dr John Taylor

INTRODUCTION

There are so many beautiful times in our lives when we feel so free and happy to Live freely as humans and enjoy the beauty of the outside world but that smell coming out of our legs has decided to become a hindrance to our social life and exposure. You want to take off your shoes and sit down on the couch with your legs moving freely but you just can't. This is not because you are an introvert, or you enjoy staying on your own and staying away from the things available in the outside world but its all because of one personal reason or should we call it a problem which is known as smelly feet.

Your feet smell so bad, and the odour makes you feel so uncomfortable and sometimes sad. Remember when you wanted to go out on that date or that meeting or should I say that event which would have added a lot of positive value to your life but you had to cancel the date, you had to postpone the meeting without a genuine reason, you lied to family and friends and refused to see them just because you don't want them you perceive the bad odour coming out from your feet. I know how you feel, and I want to make you understand that its just temporary and you can solve and will solve this problem after reading the content in this book.

We both know you are not a dirty person; you take good care of yourself and you always make sure you put things in other but there are somethings which you skipped on daily basis and these things are the reason why your feet smell in a bad way. Believe me when I tell you that you are not the only one, there are lots of people facing this same situation round the world and they are all asking the same question everyday which I am sure you have also asked yourself this question which goes like this "How can I stop my feet from having this odour". This answer to this question and the solution to this problem is in this book and I am glad that you are ready to solve the problem and get back to your best mood as a person.

I would advise that you should place your mind that you are ready to act because that is the second step after reading this book. You need to understand that even if you have the solution to the problem, you are facing but you don't act, your feet will remain the same way and you will get no results.

Chapter 1

What are smelly feet?

Smelly feet are a medical condition that includes having a solid and terrible smell from the two feet which causes you to feel awkward in broad daylight and when you remove your shoes at home. This medical condition is available among such countless individuals of any age and orientation. Have it at the back of your mind that this medical condition can't and won't kill you, yet it has a few mental and passionate impacts on the existence of an individual. There are days when this awful stench can kill your trust in broad daylight and cause you to feel deterred to engage in the things which you like to do once you are together with your loved ones.

In the clinical line, Smelly feet are called Bromodosis. The terrible smell coming from our legs can be a result of the kind of skin we have or our everyday schedule and exercises as people.

Have it at the back of your mind that this medical condition can't and won't kill you

One thing I have seen or found out with regards to individuals with smelly feet is that they find it difficult to discuss their condition and this makes them keep it hidden and consequently, it just deteriorates as time goes on. I once had a friend a very long time in the college who had a skin-related issue which he would continuously mind his own business. Whenever we shook hands, I would see his palms were so wet and doused with water. I would ask him for what valid reason his hands were so wet and cold; however, he would let me know he went to clean up certain minutes prior and I accepted. On a specific day, I went to his place of home unsuspecting when I got in, I found his home was having a horrible smell which was coming from his shoes and socks. He was experiencing sweat-soaked feet and palms, yet he never discussed it openly. This in the end pushed me to begin making research on the best way to tackle this issue on sweat-soaked feet and rank feet.

In this aide, I will be offering to you the right information which you can use to tackle the Smelly feet issues which you have been facing. I will disclose to you the causes, the answer for this issue, and how you can keep this issue from repeating later. The beautiful piece of this guide is, you would do every one of these from the comfort of your home, and you will spend a tiny sum in obtain your outcomes.

Chapter 2

Features of the human foot and smelly feet.

The human foot has a main role which incorporates conveying the heaviness of an individual and moving from one destination to another. The foot can be isolated into three areas: the forefoot, midfoot, and hindfoot. There are bones, joints, muscles, ligaments, and tendons in every one of these areas. The human foot is a solid and complex mechanical design containing 26 bones,33 joints (20 of which are effectively expressed), and more than 100 muscles, ligaments, and tendons.

The human foot is covered with skin and sweat organs. The skin is apparent so anyone might see for themselves however our perspiration organs are not noticeable like the skin. Sweat organs are little, curled, simple rounded organs that produce sweat. The skin on the two feet has an aggregate of 250,000 organs which makes around one cup of sweat day by day. This implies the human feet can deliver more perspiration than some other piece of the body.

> The human foot is covered with skin and sweat organs

You could say this isn't accurate on the grounds that you think you sweat more on your armpits and your back yet I'm here to let you that know if you focus on your entire body, you will see that your feet bring out more sweat than your armpits.

Bromodosis (Smelly feet) doesn't simply happen in hot weather. Your feet sweat consistently, regardless the temperature might be on that day. While anybody can get stinky feet, it's assessed that 10% to 15% surprisingly have feet that are smellier than normal. These individuals have a certain bacteriumon their feet called Kyetococcus sedentarius that makes sulfuric mixtures. These mixtures can make sweat smell like spoiled eggs. You need to understand that this is not a disease but a condition which can be taken care of and prevented.

Certain individuals are bound to have sweat-soaked feet. For instance, ladies and youngsters might get sweatier because of hormonal changes in their bodies. Individuals with hyperhidrosis may likewise have sweatier feet since this condition causes abundance sweating. Thusly, the additional perspiration can make your feet smell horrible prompting nasal discomfort.

Chapter 3

Causes of smelly feet.

In this section, I will clarify and make you understand the significant reasons for Smelly Feet. The recorded causes are the things that cause your feet to develop that scent that you perceive at whatever point you remove your shoes.

Presence of Bacteria and Fungus on the feet.

Bacteria are also responsible for smelly feet. Bacteria are single-celled creatures that are basically all over: in the ground, in the sea, on your hands, and in your throat. While some are destructive, a few Bacteria are not unsafe, and some are even gainful to human wellbeing. People keep a commonly advantageous connection with microscopic organisms without knowing it.

> These Bacteria live off the perspiration that your feet are continually delivering

There are numerous sorts of Bacteria on the lower part of your feet, and they reach out to your feet when your feet get filthy or sweat-soaked. These Bacteria live off the perspiration that your feet are continually delivering. Whenever they feed on the perspiration, the Bacteria make a corrosive that causes foot scent. Other than Bacteria, Fungus may likewise make you have smelly feet. Fungus develops and flourishes in warm, damp regions. Whenever your feet sweat inside your shoes and socks, this establishes an environment where fungus can grow.

Consistent Sweating of the feet.

Most times we end up participating in exercises that requires us to move from our place to one more in harsh and sunny weather. Because of these activities and movement, we sweat a lot, and our feet are not forgotten about. Many people sweat more on their feet than other parts of their body, yet they don't have any idea, and they are not attentive on the grounds that they put on socks and shoes day by day. Our socks and shoes take in the smell from our feet when we sweat on occupied days, most particularly working hours.

Many people sweat more on their feet than other parts of their body

In the clinical area, extreme sweating additionally has a name called Hyperhidrosis. Hyperhidrosis, otherwise called polyhidrosis or sudorrhea, is a condition described by excessive sweating. The sweating can influence only one region or the entire body. I have seen individuals who sweat on their palms, their backs, their necks, on their appearances, on their pubic regions, and their feet, Indeed, their feet. At the point when we sweat on our feet, we accept it as nothing on the grounds that shortly the sweats get and dried up by our socks and shoe, since that solitary impact the human feet start to develop an exceptionally awful and awkward smell which turns out to be extremely disappointing to our nose and the weather.

Dry Dead Skins on the feet.

Having dry, harsh, or broke skin on the feet is normal among people. The feet have less oil organs than different region of the body, and they experience everyday wear and tear. These dry skins are glaring to such an extent that the second you remove your shoes, you would feel the unpleasant surface around your feet which could likewise be broken with lines and occasionally become wounds on the feet. Dry skin frequently shows up on the impact points and sides of the feet and between the toes. It could cause the impacted region to feel itchy, tight, and surprisingly painful over the long run. People of all gender and ages can have dead dry skin and there are various reasons for this dry dead skin.

It could cause the impacted region to feel itchy, tight, and surprisingly painful over the long run

Absence of moisture is a significant reason for dry dead skin. At the point when oil is missing on that region of the skin, the skin starts to get very dry over the long run. Wearing inadequately fitted shoes and overabundance hotness can aggravate the skin which would prompt the harsh and broke surface on your skin. . The type of soap you use while bathing also plays a huge role on your skin surface, a few soaps can cause dry skin and make your feet look so white and cracked after having your shower.

You will see this when you sit tight for a couple of moments after having your bath, and you don't rub cream or lotion on your skin. Finally, your age can likewise cause dry dead skin. The older you become the more vulnerable your skin turns into; this is a characteristic and steady change in each human.

Dirty and Thick Socks.

A significant number of us are at real fault when it comes to putting on thick socks because of the exquisite plans and how firm they hold our legs prior to placing in our shoes. These thick socks were made with synthetic materials which restrict airflow on our feet. In a circumstance where you wind up in a stuffy and high-temperature weather, you start to sweat on your feet and your thick socks soaks this perspiration, and it would start to develop an awful scent when you don't wash your socks after use.

> Bacteria occurs and breeds on that socks when they are not washed after use

Many individuals are at real fault for not washing their socks after multiple usage. They save the used socks in a crate for a long time without washing the thick socks. Recollect these socks have been soaked before by sweat following a difficult day. Bacteria occurs and breeds on that socks when they are not washed after use. Having Bacteria on your feet is an essential piece of your body's wellbeing however it tends to be reduced when we make some private life changes like washing our socks following use. You can go 100% of the time for socks that are not excessively thick, socks that are light and can take in air which will lessen the hot temperature on the feet and decrease the degree of sweat on the feet.

Ignoring Foot Care.

It's exceptionally normal for individuals to ignore their foot wellbeing until they're experiencing severe pain or odour. The issue with neglecting your feet is it could prompt more significant issues that could affect the other parts of your body. A few activities might be hurtful to others since they are highly infectious. Individuals think when you talk about foot care, you are referring to some expensive session at the spar which isn't accurate.

It's exceptionally normal for individuals to ignore their foot wellbeing

There are basic home foot care strategies that are exceptionally useful and successful to people overall. I consider them the “Do it yourself” procedures. These methods incorporate soaking your feet regularly with clean and warm water. This can help your feet, yet your general wellbeing by loosening up muscles, diminishing pain, and bringing down pressure. After soaking your feet, utilize a straight edge toenail trimmer to cut nails straight across, which keeps away from agonizing ingrown toenails, then file your toenails with an emery board to smooth the edges.

Try not to walk shoeless ever, particularly at the exercise center. Ensure you put on your soft snickers at the gym. Change your socks as often as possible and ensure your shoe is appropriately fitted to your foot, when shoes are too large it causes people to accommodate the improper fit in a weird way.

Like I said before, these are basic and powerful foot care which you can serenely do all alone. You needn't bother with a specialist or a Masseuse to do these little practices for you. You decide immediately, and you can start from today to take great and individual consideration of your feet. Trust me, you would see positive changes.

Chapter 4

Psychological effects caused by smelly feet to a person.

Besides the physical effects we encounter as humans when it comes to having smelly feet, we also encounter and suffer some mental or psychological effect too. There are certain times in your life when you go out with friends or you find yourself in public places, you feel so free and confident when communicating with people and engaging in different activities publicly because you are clean, and you smell nice. We should look at this scenario in the contrary circumstance, I mean a circumstance where there is a smell emerging from your foot and unfortunately the following individual sitting near you can likewise perceive this awful scent coming from your feet. This will kill your confidence level in open social events and cause you to feel less good when you are amidst individuals.

This will kill your confidence level in open social events and cause you to feel less good when you are amidst individuals.

Consequently, this will lessen your degree of communication and commitment in different exercises now. This is one major issue that individuals with rancid feet face in the public arena. This will in general push them inside and makes them won't participate in other outer exercises which will influence their human relationship and their effect outwardly world. I once had a friend in those days in school, he was always quick to run back home immediately after school. I saw this attitude and ask him for what good reason he doesn't participate in other school exercises; he would cover it up saying he had activities at home and that was the justification for why he was dependably in a hurry home day by day after school. Thus, on a specific day, I chose to go visit him after school without letting him know. When I got to his home, I knocked on his door and I was astonished it took him over three minutes before he opened the door for me to come in.

Getting into his room I saw there was an awful smell in his room, it was awful to the point that I needed to ask him right away assuming this was the if this was the reason why he was always running home after school. He opened up to me saying "I have been living with this horrible smell for a long time and I don't have the any idea on how to stop it. I understood he had sweat-soaked feet's and he was aware 100% at that time of his current circumstance, so others won't take note.

This smell has impacted his communication level and impacted his confidence level personally. He finds it difficult to relate with others since he feels they will see the terrible stench and avoid him. He decided to remain alone and drive away the rest of the world and its exercises. At that point I realized he really wanted an answer for his problem, and he really wanted it rapidly. We began by discarding every one of the thick socks and dirty socks in his room. Then, at that point, we moved to different arrangements which could be valuable in assisting him with solving the terrible smell and bring back his confidence level. These solutions will be completely clarified in the following part of this book.

Chapter 5

How to stop your feet from smelling bad.

I realize this is the part you have been sitting tight for right from the second you started reading this book. In this part, I will be thoroughly clarifying ways and systems which will assist you with totally preventing your feet from having that terrible scent.

Washing Your Feet with Anti Bacteria Soaps.

Antibacterial soaps are brands of soap or cleansers that contain chemical ingredients that have a major goal which is helping with killing Bacteria and different germs on the human body. Antibacterial soaps (now and again called antimicrobial or antiseptic soaps) contain specific synthetic compounds not found in plain soaps. Those ingredients are added to numerous anti bacteria soaps with the goal of decreasing or forestalling bacterial contamination.

> You should wash your skin with the antibacterial two times every day

How do you tell if a product (Soap) is antibacterial? For OTC medications, antibacterial items by and large have "antibacterial" on the mark. Likewise, also, a Drug Facts label on a soap or body wash is a sign a product contains antibacterial ingredients. Antibacterial soaps and handwashes are utilized broadly in the home, work environment, childcare and medical services conditions, and occupations connected with food arrangement in the conviction they are more effective than ordinary soaps and water at at preventing illness and reducing the transmission of bacteria contamination. There are manners by which you can utilize these antibacterial cleansers and they will not be destructive to your skin. You should wash your skin with the antibacterial two times every day (Morning and Evening) yet assuming you have a smelly foot that you're desire to solve its advisable you use the soap to wash your feet immediate you get home and take off your socks and shoes.

Place your feet under or in warm water for around three to four minutes, then, at that point, rub the two feet gradually with the anti-bacteria soap and ensure it contacts all region of your feet, do this consistently until you are certain the soap is on each region of your foot. The following stage is scrubbing your feet either utilizing your hands, a wipe, or gentle body clean towel. Scrub all region of your feet and do it for a few minutes. Ensure you are Scrubbing tenderly and not excessively cruel, so you won't hurt your feet or cause any injury because of forceful cleaning. The cleaning process will eliminate and lessen the bacterial level on your feet and keep it spotless and smooth.

In the wake of cleaning, you should flush your feet with clean water and cold water. The flushing will remove the soap from your feet alongside the Bacteria which has been taken out by the soap and water from your feet. Try not to utilize heated water while washing your feet and don't rush this cycle so you won't miss a few places where the Bacteria could stow away. In the wake of washing then you should pass on your feet to dry all alone or you can utilize a spotless dry towel to dry your feet. Recall that I said a spotless dry towel.

Do not wear the same shoes for two days in a row and for long hours.

We all have that unique and most loved shoe which we love to put on for occasions and events. Whenever you put on that shoe, we you often look more alluring, tasteful and it expands our classy and it increases our level of confidence in the public. We frequently put on this shoe with our socks two times or multiple times in succession in multi week and we feel it's alright and great practice. This is one of the significant reasons for smelly feet and even though it very well may be difficult for you to stop this training, you simply should stop it assuming you want to have a foot that doesn't smell or create a terrible scent openly. You need to get used to keeping your beloved shoe to the side for certain days and set on different shoes at whatever point you are taking off for work or an occasion. Rotating your shoes can help them last longer and make your feet to have an improved outlook.

Rotating your shoes can help them last longer and make your feet to have an improved outlook.

A significant justification for why you really want to change or turn your shoes every day is that our feet get splashed over the course of the day and when they get drenched, it influences the shoes by making them doused as well and its best for you to take out time the following day to dry your shoes before you wear them for the following occasion.

Wearing cleans soft socks before putting on your shoe.

The type of socks, you put on day by day assumes a huge part in the state of your feet personally. These socks are of various lengths, materials, and colors in the marketplace. We wear socks to shield our feet from having rankles, shoe nibbles and to make our shoes fit flawlessly. The sort of socks we have includes the High Socks/Over the Knee Socks, the Knee Socks, the Calf Socks, the Mid-Calf Socks, the Lower leg Socks and the Flake-out Socks. These Socks are worn at various seasons and for various events.

We wear socks to shield our feet from having rankles, shoe nibbles and to make our shoes fit flawlessly.

Continuously ensure your socks are perfect and guarantee you buy short socks with a delicate material on the off chance that if you are the type of person who sweats a lot on your feet. These sorts of socks will help in expanding the degree of wind current into your point of view and will decrease the degree of sweating that you experience day by day. Always remember to separate your clean and dry socks according to their colors to avoid confusion the next time you want to put them on for that special occasion.

Spray your feet with Anti-Perspirant sprays daily.

Antiperspirant is a skincare item that lessens underarm sweating and the feet of an individual. This isn't to be mistaken for deodorant, which is just there to battle and remove the terrible scent. Antiperspirants work by obstructing the pores on the external layer of your skin, decreasing how much perspiration permitted to the surface. With a good Anti-Perspirant spray, you can lessen the undeniable degree of steady sweating on your feet and feel better while wearing your socks and shoes. Aluminium salts are included in antiperspirants to help reduce the sweat flow in the underarm region. The salts restrict access to the upper part of the sweat glands so that it is more difficult for sweat to be released. Deodorants are totally different from Anti-Perspirant Spray in the sense that one fights bad odour and the other blocks the sweat pores and reduces the high level of sweating on that area of the skin.

> With a good Anti-Perspirant spray, you can lessen the undeniable degree of steady sweating on your feet and feel better while wearing your socks and shoes

Using an Anti-Perspirant Spray is very easy, yet you can likewise fail to understand the situation if you don't follow the instructions. In the first place, you want to scrub down or shower, then, at that point, you clean the region of the foot with a spotless and dry towel. After cleaning the feet, ensure your feet are dried totally then you shake the anti-perspirant spray and hold it around 15 cm away from your feet and the Shower straightforwardly on the feet. Do this every day before leaving home. Do not spray on your face or directly to your eye because it could damage your sight and send you straight to the hospital.

Use Apple Juice Vinegar to wash your feet.

Apple cider vinegar is mostly apple juice, but adding yeast turns the sugar in the juice into alcohol. This is a process called fermentation. Bacteria turn the alcohol into acetic acid. That gives vinegar its sharp taste and solid smell which makes you want to puke or throw up when you perceive an original Vinegar. Apple juice vinegar has a long history as a home cure, used to deal with things like sore throat and varicose veins even though there isn't a lot of science that supports these claims. Vinegar is utilized in cooking, baking, and salad dressings and as an additive. There's a great deal of acid in it, so drinking vinegar straight isn't suggested.

It can create some issues, such as disintegrating the polish of your teeth, assuming you get excessively. Yet, as of late, a few scientists have been investigating apple juice vinegar and its potential advantages, they found it can likewise be utilized to treat smelly feet and eliminate bacteria from the feet of an individual. Vinegar has been utilized as a solution for hundreds of years. Historians have likewise spread the word about it that the ancient Greeks treated injuries with Apple Juice Vinegar.

Vinegar has been utilized as a solution for hundreds of years

Apple juice vinegar has the antimicrobial potential to assist with killing Bacteria and with it the scent. Absorbing your feet an answer of 1/3 cup of apple juice vinegar in a bowl of water could assist with disposing of the smell. Because of apple juice vinegar's antibacterial properties, it can assist with killing the scent causing Bacteria on your feet. While it's generally expected and sound that your body is covered with a variety of microscopic organisms and different Bacteria altogether called the skin microbiome at times that Bacteria can escape balance. Then when your body produces sweat, the bacteria overgrowth "feeds" on the sweat and produces pungent, less-than-ideal smells. Apple cider vinegar has also been shown to have antiviral, anti-yeast, and antifungal benefits, all helpful in supporting your microbiome balance. In a study, scientists found that the vinegar can inhibit growth of C. albicans in a petri dish. It works by destroying the fungus' cell structure, along with specific enzymes the fungus needs to survive. Before soaking your feet in Apple Cider Vinegar, make sure you thoroughly wash your legs with an anti-bacteria soap and water. Do this twice or three times a week and do not let the soaking exceed 15 minutes at max.

www.ingramcontent.com/pod-product-compliance
Ingram Content Group UK Ltd.
Pitfield, Milton Keynes, MK11 3LW, UK
UKHW022009190726
13853UKWH00004B/1826

9 798421 573432